First published 2019

www.books.wellstore.ng

CONTENT

INTRODUCTION

Women...... caring for everyone else but self!

This guide written in simple terms will educate women about their bodies and how to take charge of their health and wellbeing. It contains useful information on self-care, warning signals and routine screening to ensure a healthy, balanced life.

Now, equipped with this information, women can become partners in the management of their health.

All information provided are based on scientific research and established facts and has been reviewed by qualified health professionals.

CHAPTER 1

AN AMAZING BODY

A middle-aged woman walked into the clinic looking worried.

Patient: Hello Doctor, I noticed some redness in my private part two days ago.

Doctor: where exactly is the redness?

Patient: in my private part she repeated, already getting impatient.

The Doctor must perform a quick examination to identify the affected area. Care for the body starts with knowing its structure and function. It is so important to be able to identify your body parts as a woman.

THE FEMALE BODY

The female body is simply incredible. From structure to function, it is unique in all aspects. One of the most startling questions in the Holy Writ is; "Do you know how bones grow in the womb?" Think about it! Think of a body that can grow another human being, bring it forth and then feed it, awesome!

It's time to get down to the basics of identifying the female body parts.

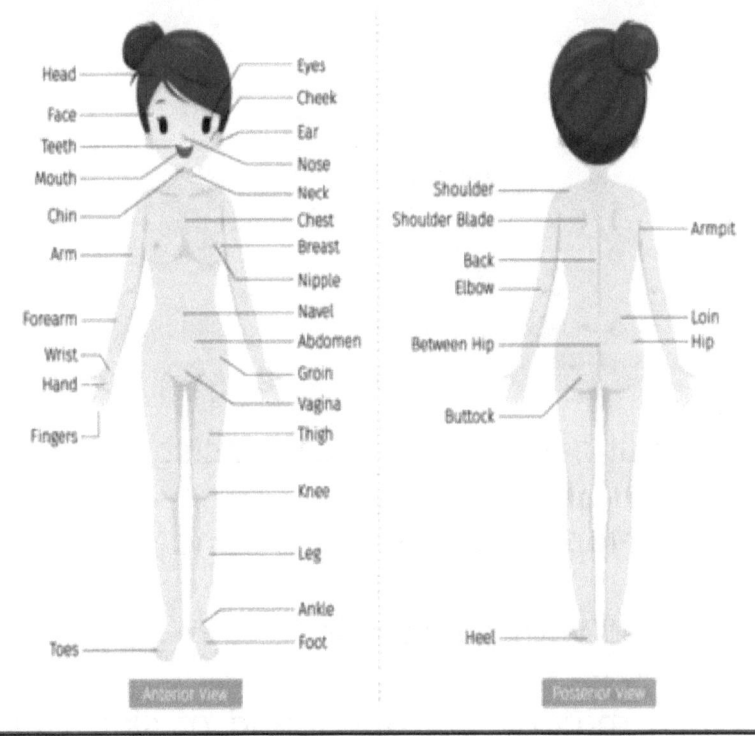

Diagram 1

THE FEMALE REPRODUCTIVE SYSTEM

This comprises of organs which function in producing offspring. The organs in the female reproductive system is broadly divided into the external and internal reproductive organs.

External Genitals

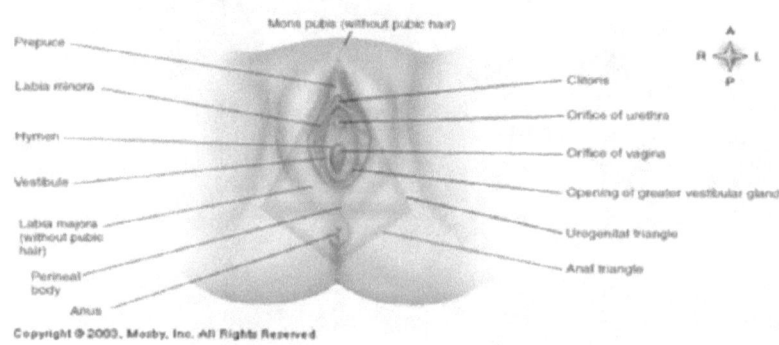

The external genitalia (Vulva) consist of

- The Mons pubis- A mound of tissue covered with pubic hair.

- Labia majora- An outer fold of skin (outer lip)

- Labia minora- An inner fold of skin (inner lip)
- Vestibule- The part between the labia minora which has two openings: the urethral and vaginal opening.
- The Clitoris: A small structure at the bottom of the mons pubis, covered by the labia minora.

The hymen is a thin membrane across the vaginal opening. It undergoes partial rupture during first coitus

(Sex) and is further disrupted during childbirth.

Note: The hymen may be ruptured due to physical activities such as exercise. Its absence does not exclude virginity.

INTERNAL REPRODUCTIVE ORGANS

This consists of

- The Vagina: A muscular tube which connects with the cervix.

- The Uterus (Womb): This is an elastic structure that receives a fertilized egg and accommodates a developing fetus.

  It is divided into two parts:

  Body- This is the upper part.

  Cervix- This is the lower part which connects to the vagina.

- The fallopian tubes- These are fine tubes that transport mature egg from the ovary to the uterus.

- The ovaries- These are organs that produce eggs and secrete hormones which regulate reproductive processes.

There are also organs that are closely related such as:

- The bladder: A temporary store for urine.
- The Ureters: Thin tubes connecting the kidneys to the bladder, and transports urine produced by the kidneys to the bladder for storage.
- The Urethra: Short tube that allows flow of urine from the bladder.
- The urethral opening is below the clitoris in females and discharges urine.

- The Rectum: The part of the large intestine that temporarily stores faeces.

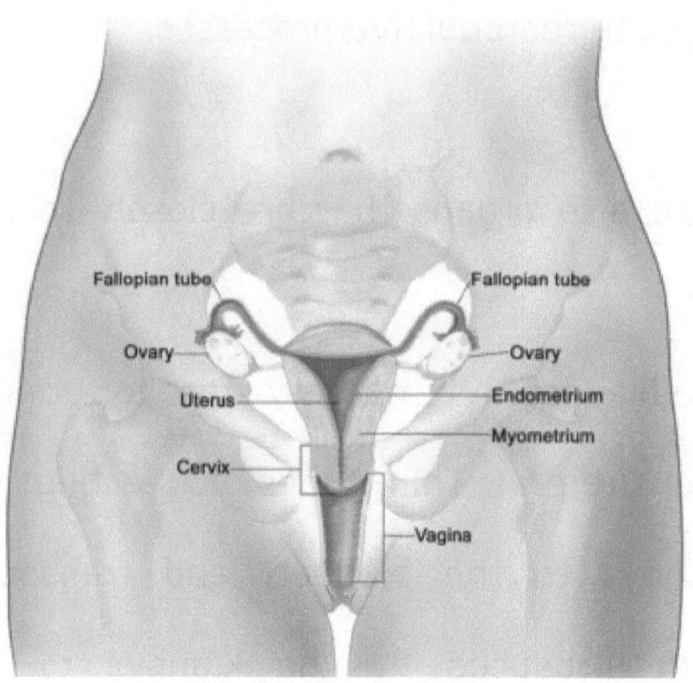

FACTS ABOUT THE FEMALE BODY

FACTS ABOUT THE FEMALE BODY

- The uterus (womb) is ultra elastic.

- The vagina is acidic.

- No woman has equal sized breasts.

- The ovaries have numerous eggs, capable of becoming a fetus and all are present at birth.
- The clitoris is solely for pleasure.

CHAPTER 2

THE BREAST

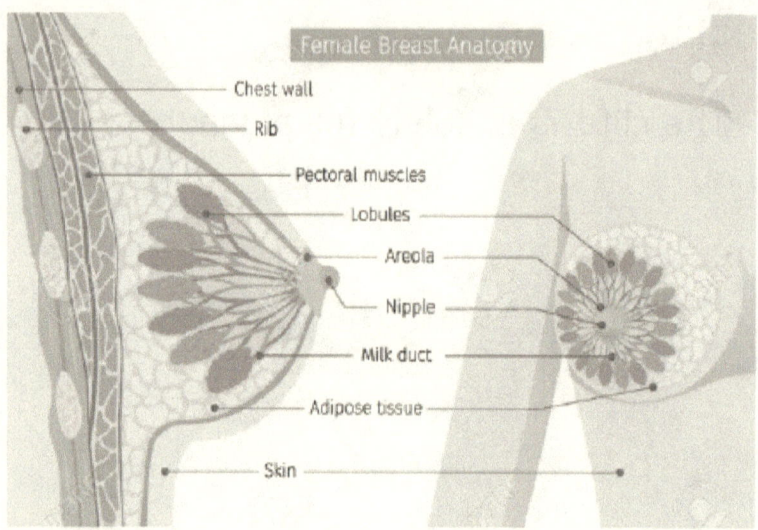

Diagram 1

The female breast is undoubtedly one attractive feature of the female body; beautiful structure, awesome function.

Breasts consist of skin, glandular tissue, connective tissue, ductal lobule units, ligaments, and fat. While breasts are always changing, they're not considered completely mature until pregnancy or lactation occurs.

"The ductal lobule units don't get mature until they get the signal of lactation, or sometimes they just give up and fully mature about two years after onset of menstruation," says Amanda wheeler, MD, breast surgeon at Stanford Health Care and clinical assistant professor of surgery at the Stanford University School of Medicine in California.

Once women enter the perimenopausal years — usually in their forties — changes that lead to sagging occur. "The ductal lobule units will no longer be supported by hormones. When that happens, they shrivel up and shrink, with fatty replacement of the breast," Dr. Wheeler explains. "Plus, as women age, connective tissue, which suspends the breasts up and acts as a natural underwear of the breast, gets stretched. The breast skin begins to lose elasticity too, and both contribute to sagging."

FACTS ABOUT THE BREAST

1. It is normal to have a slight difference in size between both breasts. No two breasts are alike, even on the same person, says Wheeler. "While a woman's nipples and areolas tend to be consistent on both breasts, one breast is usually larger than the other."

However, significant difference in size should be a cause for concern. Other differences may include one being higher or rounder than the other.

2. Breast milk is real meal

Breast milk can sustain a baby for up to six months without additional food or water. The breast has the capacity to produce enough milk to meet this demand. It is also good to know that a woman can breastfeed while pregnant.

3. The breast gives out smell.

Montgomery glands (Little bumps around the areola) give out scent that smells like amniotic fluid that only babies can detect.

4. Most breast lumps are discovered by women.

Women can detect slight changes in breast tissue and more so during self-examination.

6. Not all lumps are cancerous:

Most breast lumps are not cancer, according to the American Cancer Society. Rather, the most common types of lumps are fibrosis, cysts (fluidfilled sacs), and other non-cancerous or benign breast tumors. A swollen, painful lump may be a breast abscess, or collection of pus caused by an infection.

7. The risk of breast cancer increases with age

Yes! with age, a woman becomes more at risk for breast cancer. However it can be treated if detected early.

BREAST SELF-EXAMINATION

Self-examination of the breast will help detect lumps and other abnormalities early. This is easy to do!

WHEN?

It should be done monthly, few days after menstruation.

Menopausal women can choose a particular date each month.

HOW?

STEP 1:

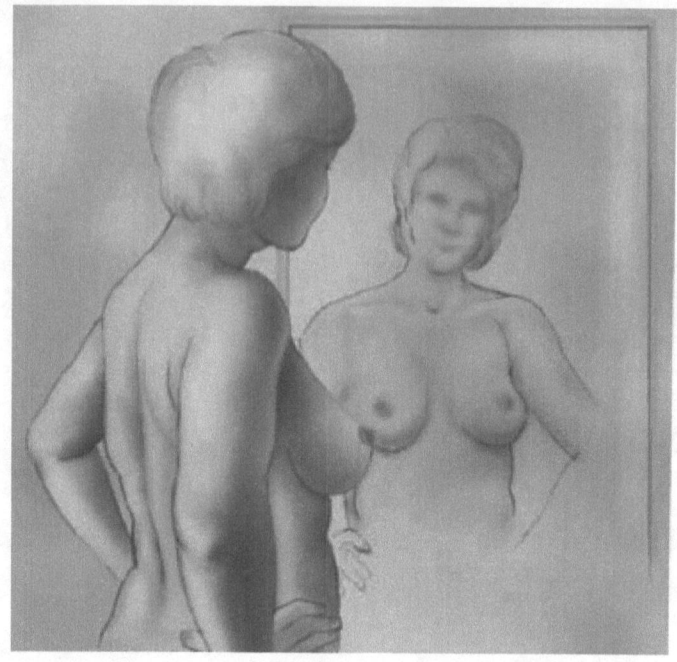

Stand in front of a mirror with hands on your hips and inspect both breasts.

Check for:

1. Change in size, shape or position of entire breast.

2. Change in nipple shape or position.

3. Change in skin over the breast such as redness, dimpling.

STEP 2:

Place your arms over your head and inspect again.

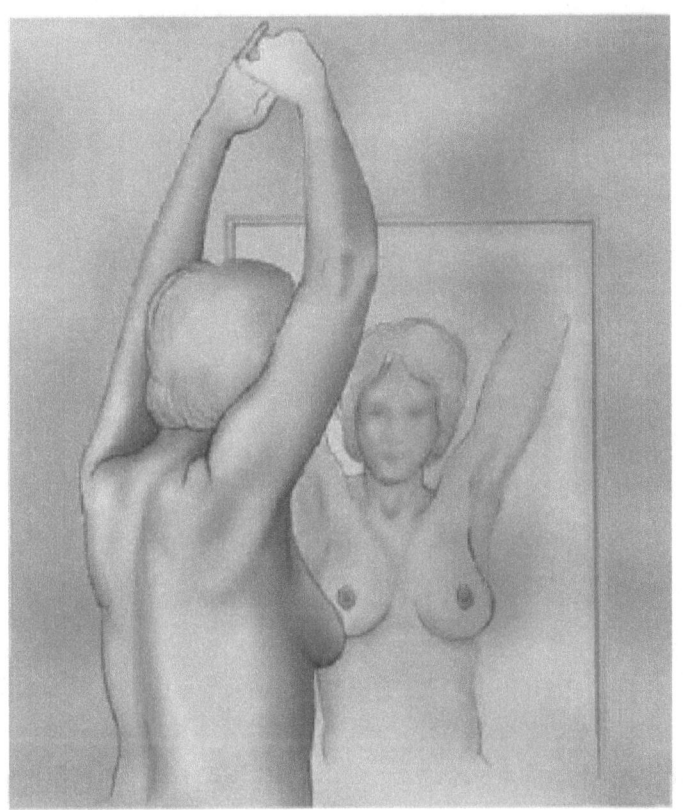

STEP 3:

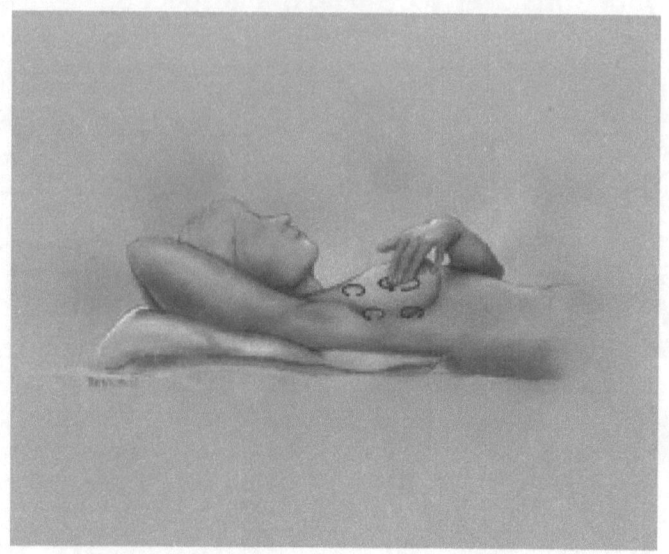

1. Lie flat, placing one arm over your head. With the other hand, massage all regions of the breast in a spiral pattern, beginning from the nipple area. Do not forget to check the axilla (armpit) area.

2. Gently squeeze the nipples to check for discharge.

STEP 4: Repeat step 3 while sitting or standing.

STEP 5: Record your findings.

WARNING SIGNALS:

- Lump

- Nipple discharge

- Change in shape of breast/ nipple

- Pain

- Redness, itchiness, rash

- Dimpling of the skin.

- Visible veins on the breast

- Nodes in the armpit.

BREAST HEALTH TIPS

I. Do breast self-examination monthly and a professional breast examination yearly.

II. Wear clean, well-fitting bra.

III. Avoid harmful chemicals in personal care products such as Aluminum salts in deodorants, parabens in body lotion etc.

IV. Breastfeed babies for as long as possible. This reduces the risk of developing breast cancer.

V. Do a mammogram every other year from the age of 40years.

CONFIDENT VAGINA

The vagina is a muscular, elastic canal that extends from the cervix to the hymen. Many use the term vagina colloquially to encompass all parts of the female genitalia. Technically, the vulva is the term that should be used to refer to the external female sex organs, including the clitoris, urethra, the labia majora and minora (outer and inner vaginal lips respectively), and the mons pubis.

The vagina is kept moist by mucus produced in the cervix.

FUNCTIONS OF THE VAGINA

For coitus (sex).

An outlet for menstrual blood.

Birth canal.

CARE OF THE VAGINA

A healthy vagina is important to a woman's overall health and well-being.

Note: The vagina needs little care as it has a self-cleaning

WARNING SIGNALS

I. Change in color, odour or amount of vaginal discharge.

II. Redness

III. Itchiness

IV. Abnormal bleeding

V. pain

VI. Growth.

VAGINAL HEALTH TIPS

- Practice safe sex

- Get vaccinations e.g. HPV (Human Papilloma Virus) vaccination. Human papilloma virus is implicated in most cases of cervical cancer.

- Do not douche- douching involves washing out the vagina with water or other substances.

- Wash vulva and external genitalia such as the labia to get rid of build-up of oils and dead skin hidden in the folds.

- Wear well-fitting cotton pants.

- Do not use soap, perfumes or spray on vaginal tissue.

- Avoid use of scented pads and tampons

- Shave with a fresh, clean razor blade.

- Use water based lubricants during sex to increase lubrication and avoid micro-tears which can become infected.

- Urinate after sex and practice washing from front to back

- Air the vagina. Vagina also needs fresh air to breathe. Go underwear free once in a while and during sleep.

- Take foods rich in probiotics such as yoghurt to maintain the vagina's natural bacteria and reduce the risk of yeast infection.

- Do kegel's exercise regularly to strengthen muscles of the pelvic floor which supports the vagina.

- Practice self-examination using a mirror to look out for changes in the vagina.

FACTS ABOUT THE VAGINA

1. Pubic hair has a purpose.

Before making the shave (or going full-on with laser hair removal or waxing), it's good to know that pubic hair has a job. Specifically, it "serves as a protective barrier to genital tissues, particularly the sensitive vaginal opening. As well as providing a protective barrier, it also acts as a buffer against friction.

Shaving can leave tiny wounds (microtears) on the skin, temporarily increasing one's risk of infection.

2. Discharge is usually normal, but not always.

The quality and quantity of cervical fluid changes throughout a cycle, and are responses to the hormonal transitions that prepare the body for ovulation, explain Högemann and Druet. "Cervical fluid starts opaque, whitish, and creamy during early follicular phase— around the start of a cycle," they say. "It increases in quantity, wetness, transparency, and stretchiness as ovulation approaches. Cervical fluid reaches peak characteristics of fertility around the day of ovulation, which include a wet, clear, and stretchy texture."

3. The vagina is self-cleaning.

The lining of the vagina is made up of various glands that release fluids designed to cleanse and lubricate the vagina. The use of soap will always interfere with the vagina's natural bacterial flora, which can upset the body's pH balance and cause infections, such as candidiasis (thrush). Soap should not be used anywhere beyond the outermost labia, where pubic hair grows.

Douching, which is the rinsing of the vagina with vinegar or an antiseptic with the aid of a douche bag, can increase the risk of vaginal and pelvic infection by altering the pH and ridding the vagina of important bacteria. Research shows a link between douching and increasing the risk of bacterial vaginosis, pelvic inflammatory infections, and ectopic pregnancy.

4. The vagina does change, especially after childbirth.

The cervical opening may change slightly in appearance—from a dot to more of a curve—but it is still closed and fulfills the same purpose. While vaginal tissue stretches during labor, it should return to its same size without much intervention.

5. Kegels are basically "vaginal anti-aging creams."

Dr. Gerber recommends every woman practice Kegel exercises after a vaginal birth, following a doctor's clearance. "The way women use wrinkle creams, everyone should be doing Kegels. And definitely after childbirth," she says. To properly locate the muscles, Dr. Gerber suggests a technique one of her mentors taught her: "Pretend that you're in an elevator, and you need to pass gas, but you are trying to prevent it." That way, you'll activate all of the muscles in the pelvic floor, she says.

6. After birth, vaginas need a rest.

Whether it's a vaginal birth or a C-section, doctors advise women to avoid penetration for six weeks after giving birth, as the vagina needs that time to heal.

7. Vaginas are 'Acidic'

Vaginas have an acid environment with a pH level of 4.5, which allows sperm to swim and survive once inside.

8. They come in all different colours.

Labia colour can range from light pink to dark brown. During sexual arousal, the colour of the labia can temporarily deepen as blood rushes to the area.

9. No two vaginas smell the same.

So many different factors go into a woman's southern scent. Every woman smells a slightly different, thanks to her diet, the fabric she wears, her gland secretions, level of hygiene and her personal blend of internal bacteria.

REPRODUCTIVE HEALTH

The female body is complex in structure and function. Reproductive health refers to conditions that affect the functioning of the reproductive system. Good sexual and reproductive health is a state of complete physical, mental and social well-being in all matters relating to the reproductive system. It implies that people are able to have a satisfying and safe sex life, the capability to reproduce, and the freedom to decide if, when, and how often to do so.

Reproductive health of women is very important as it affects general health and wellbeing.

Different stages of a woman's life are associated with specific sexual and reproductive health issues, including menstruation, fertility, cervical screening, contraception, pregnancy, sexually transmissible infections, chronic health problems (such as endometriosis and polycystic ovary syndrome) and menopause.

THE MENSTRUAL CYCLE

Menstruation, also called menses is the discharge of blood and tissue from the uterus, through the vagina.

It usually happens every month.

A menstrual cycle starts from the first day of a period and ends on the first day of the next period.

The average cycle length is 28 days.

Cycle length between 21-35 days is considered normal.

Menstrual flow of 2-8days is normal.

There are three phases in the menstrual cycle. This illustration is based on a typical cycle length of 28days.

1. The Follicular Phase: this phase will last for 14 days from the first day of bleeding to the 14th day. A Period is the actual days of bleeding which last between 2 to 8 days.

2. Ovulation Phase: This is the release of a mature egg (ovum) from the ovary. This occurs

approximately on the 14th day of the follicular phase.

3. Luteal Phase: this phase will last for 14 days from the 14th to 28th day of the cycle; 14 days before the next cycle.

SIGNS OF OVULATION

Cervical mucus becomes clear, slippery and stretchy.

- Slight increase in body temperature.
- One sided pelvic pain.
- Breast pain.
- Bloating.

Note: some women may not experience some of the symptoms of ovulation.

CONCEPTION AND PREGNANCY

This is the process from fertilization of an egg to implantation, then development of an offspring. The highest chance of getting pregnant is on the days leading up to ovulation (ovary releases a mature egg); this is called fertile days. This egg lives for about a day after release and sperm can live in the uterus or fallopian tube for up to 5 days after sex. A woman can get pregnant for about six days of the menstrual cycle;

5 days before the day of ovulation and on the day of ovulation.

If pregnancy occurs, menstruation will stop and gestation period sets in which is an average of 40 weeks from the last menstrual period.

FACTS TO NOTE:

- The egg (ovum) survives for about 24hours after ovulation.

- Released sperm can survive for up to 3 to 5 days.

- Conception can take place 5days before ovulation up to 24hours after ovulation.

- Ovulation takes place 14days before the onset of the next menstrual period.

CHAPTER 3

MENOPAUSE

Menopause is the cessation of menstruation that marks the end of a woman's ability to reproduce. Menopause is a natural biological process.

Note

✗ Menopause takes place averagely between 45-55 years.

✗ Menses must be absent for at least 12 months.

✗ Menstrual period gradually gets irregular before cessation.

CAUSES OF MENOPAUSE

Menopause can result from:

1. Natural decline of reproductive hormones. Towards the late 30s, the ovaries start making less estrogen and progesterone — the hormones that regulate menstruation — and fertility declines. In the late 40s, menstrual periods may become longer or shorter, heavier or lighter, and more or less frequent, until eventually — on average, by age 51 — the ovaries stops producing eggs and menstruation stops.

2. Hysterectomy. A hysterectomy that removes the uterus but not the ovaries usually doesn't cause immediate menopause. Although the menstrual period stops, the ovaries still release eggs and produce estrogen and progesterone.

But surgery that removes both the uterus and ovaries (total hysterectomy and bilateral oophorectomy) does cause immediate menopause. In this case, menopausal signs and symptoms can be severe, as these hormonal changes occur abruptly rather than over several years.

3. Chemotherapy and radiation therapy. These cancer therapies can induce menopause, causing symptoms such as hot flushes during or shortly after the course of treatment. The halt to menstruation (and fertility) is not always permanent following chemotherapy, so birth control measures may still be desired.

4. Primary ovarian insufficiency. About 1 percent of women experience menopause

before age 40 (premature menopause). Menopause may result from primary ovarian insufficiency — when the ovaries fail to produce normal levels of reproductive hormones — stemming from genetic factors or autoimmune disease. But often no cause can be found. For these women, hormone therapy is typically recommended at least until the natural age of menopause in order to protect the brain, heart and bones.

SYMPTOMS OF MENOPAUSE

Menopause comes along with a myriad of symptoms, some quite overwhelming.

1. Hot flushes.

2. Night sweat.

3. Weight gain.

4. Problems with sleep.

5. Problems with memory.

6. Mood change (anxiety, depression, irritability).

7. Changes in sex drive (may increase or decrease).

8. Skin changes e.g. dry skin.

9. Itchiness/dryness of the vagina.

10. Thinning hair and dry skin.

11. Loss of breast fullness.

COMPLICATIONS OF MENOPAUSE

- After menopause, the risk of certain medical conditions increases. Examples include:

- Heart and blood vessel (cardiovascular) disease. When estrogen levels decline, the risk of cardiovascular disease increases. it's important to get regular exercise, eat a healthy diet and maintain a healthy weight.

- Osteoporosis. This condition causes bones to become brittle and weak, leading to an increased risk of fractures. During the first few years after menopause, a woman may lose bone density at a rapid rate, increasing the risk of osteoporosis.

- Postmenopausal women with osteoporosis are especially susceptible to fractures of the spine, hips and wrists.

- Urinary incontinence. As the tissues of the vagina and urethra lose elasticity, a woman may experience frequent, sudden, strong urges to urinate, followed by an involuntary loss of urine (urge incontinence), or the loss of urine with coughing, laughing or lifting (stress incontinence).

- Strengthening pelvic floor muscles with Kegel exercises and using a topical vaginal estrogen may help relieve symptoms of incontinence.

- Sexual function. Vaginal dryness from decreased moisture production and loss of elasticity can cause discomfort and slight bleeding during sexual intercourse. Also, decreased sensation may reduce the desire for sexual activity (libido). Water-based vaginal moisturizers and lubricants may help. If a vaginal lubricant isn't enough, many women benefit from the use of local vaginal estrogen treatment, available as a vaginal cream, tablet or ring.

- Weight gain. Many women gain weight during the menopausal transition and after menopause because metabolism slows. It is advisable to eat less and exercise more, to maintain weight.

COPING WITH MENOPAUSE

The key to coping with menopause is to know what to expect and how to handle it.

1. Be informed about changes associated with menopause.

2. Report any abnormality.

3. Adopt a healthy lifestyle which includes healthy diet, exercise, supplementation.

4. Keep record of symptoms.

5. Manage stress.

SPECIAL NOTE ON HOT FLUSHES

This is by far one of the most overwhelming experiences women report. It is a feeling of intense heat not due to an external source. It occurs due to hormonal changes and typically last less than five minutes.

WHAT TO DO

1. Keep the environment cool.

2. Wear loose clothing.

3. Ensure adequate intake of water.

4. Take a shower.

5. Avoid alcohol and caffeine.

CHAPTER 4

BIRTH CONTROL

Also known as contraception; it refers to any drug, device or method used to prevent pregnancy.

There are several methods of birth control ranging from Natural methods to over-the-counter products to prescription contraceptives.

Choice of a birth control product or method is dependent on the following factors:

(1) Overall Health status.

(2) Need for short or long-term contraception.

(3) The number of sex partners.

(4) personal preferences.

TYPES OF BIRTH CONTROL

1. Natural method

2. Barrier method

3. Use of Intra-uterine Device

4. Hormonal contraception

5. Sterilization

CONTRACEPTION	MODE OF ACTION	SIDE EFFECT
NATURAL METHOD	(a)RHYTHM: Abstinence from sexual intercourse during fertile period. (b)Exclusive Breastfeeding (c) Withdrawal method (coitus interruptus)	
BARRIER METHOD	Prevents direct contact of sperm and egg. **CONDOMS:-** Should be worn before any genital contact. Withdraw erect penis immediately after ejaculation	Allergy, Irritation May tear, burs t or slip off.
	DIAPHRAGM/CERVICAL CAPS: Insert immediately before intercourse.	Vaginal irritation Increased risk of urinary tract infection
INTRA-UTERINE DEVICE	Induce inflammation in the lining of the uterus to prevent implantation. E.g Copper - T	Increased risk of pelvic infection in the first few weeks. Increased menstrual flow Menstrual Pain.
HORMONAL METHOD	(A) COMBINED HORMONES; - Inhibit ovulation - Make lining of uterus hostile - Alter cervical mucus to disrupt free swimming of sperm.	- Increased risk of heart disease and breast cancer. - Weight gain irregular bleeding. - loss of libido - Headache - Bloatedness.

	(B) PROGESTERONE – ONLY (Oral, Injectable or Implant) - Make cervical mucus hostile to sperm	- Absence of menses
	- Make lining of the uterus thin to prevent implantation.	- Acne
	- Inhibit ovulation at higher doses.	- Breast pain
STERILIZATION	Blockage of both fallopian tubes to prevent sperm from reaching egg.	- Surgical complication
		- Increased risk of ectopic pregnancy.

EMERGENCY CONTRACEPTION

This refers to methods of contraception that can be used to prevent pregnancy after sexual intercourse.

Emergency contraception is recommended for use within five days of sexual exposure and are more effective the sooner they are used.

WHEN TO USE EMERGENCY CONTRACEPTION

I. Unprotected sex.

II. Failure of a barrier method e.g. burst condom.

III. Missed pill.

IV. Sexual assault if without contraceptive cover.

TYPES OF EMERGENCY CONTRACEPTION

(1) Copper-bearing Intra-uterine device (IUD).

(2) Emergency contraceptive pills (ECPs).

MODE OF ACTION:

- Copper-bearing IUD: This prevents fertilization by causing a chemical change in released sperm and egg.

- Emergency contraceptive pills prevent or delay ovulation.

SIDE EFFECT:

As in Oral contraceptive pills: Headache, nausea, vomiting, fatigue, dizziness, irregular vaginal bleeds.

NOTE

Emergency contraception pill is not an abortion pill and will not stop or harm pregnancy that has already occured.

It is not to be used as a regular birth control.

It should be used as soon as possible (best is within 72hrs) for efficacy.

FACTS ABOUT CONTRACEPTION

- Natural methods are safe, but success rate is hindered by non- compliance.

- Barrier method is suitable when preventing sexually transmitted infections e.g. in polygamous relationships.

- Insertion of Intra-uterine device must be performed by trained health care personnel and is ideal for women needing long term contraception.

- Progesterone-only pills are suitable for breastfeeding mothers and older aged women due to the absence of estrogen.

- Sterilization is a permanent method of contraception and must be carefully decided. It has a low possibility of failure.

CHAPTER 5

STAYING HEALTHY

Good health is a product of healthy habits. Now, you can take charge of your health!

HEALTHY HABITS

1. Healthy eating: a wise man once said, "Man is what he eats."

What you take in will definitely show on your skin and control your health. It is important to consider the following:

· Eat well balanced diet

· Take lots of fruits and vegetables

· Ensure adequate water intake

· Reduce fat, salt and sugar intake

· Eat lean meat

· Avoid smoking

· Limit alcohol intake

· Limit intake of processed food.

2. PHYSICAL ACTIVITY

Daily exercise improves heart health, strengthen bones and muscles.

3. BE SAFE: Practice Safe sex, keep the environment safe, engage in Safe activities.

4. Manage Stress: while stress can spur one into action, uncontrolled Stress has a negative impact on health.

5. Regular health checks: Every woman should have a doctor before she needs one. Do regular screening for common diseases. Consult with a doctor promptly for any health concern.

CHAPTER 6

KILL STRESS

Stress is the feeling of inability to cope with demands.

It could be short lived or a long time situation.

High level stress can affect one's health negatively.

TYPES OF STRESS

I. Acute stress- immediate response to a stressful situation.

II. Episodic Acute stress- when an acute stress occurs frequently.

III. Chronic stress: prolonged stress.

SYMPTOMS OF STRESS

· Irritability.

· Nervousness.

· Excessive worry.

· Sadness/ depression.

· Sleep problems.

· Change in appetite (may increase or decrease).

· Changes in libido (may increase or decrease).

· Headache.

· Infertility.

EFFECTS OF STRESS

ORGAN /SYSTEM	EFFECT
BRAIN	Headache, Irritability Anxiety Depression Insomnia
HEART	Hypertension Heart disease
DIGESTIVE	Ulcer
SKIN	Acne Eczema
REPRODUCTIVE	Inhibit ovulation
MUSCLE	Aches Twitching
LUNGS	Emotional stress can trigger Acute attacks in asthmatics
HAIR	Hair loss Thinning
IMMUNITY	Weakened

COPING WITH STRESS

I. Identify stressors and set priorities.

II. Get support from friends and family.

III. Live healthy; practice healthy eating, exercise, adequate sleep.

IV. Take breaks.

V. Be realistic in expectation of self and others.

VI. Avoid alcohol and caffeine.

VII. Be positive.

VIII. Seek medical help.

A NOTE ON SELF-NURTURING

- Women support and care for their significant other partners, kids, parents, siblings, friends and find it difficult to focus on their own needs.

Self-nurturing is important to refresh, renew and bring balance to a woman's life.

- The rule is "Do something for yourself everyday."

TIPS FOR SELF-NURTURING

Daily Meditation

Adequate Sleep

Good Nutrition

Physical Activity

SUGGESTED ACTIVITIES

- Enjoy a nice meal alone or with a loved one.

- Enjoy music and dance.

- Take a relaxing bath.

- Take a walk.

- Read uplifting literature.

- Watch a movie.

- Be kind

CHAPTER 7

HEALTHY WEIGHT

Maintaining a healthy weight improves overall health and wellbeing. The recent trend has been on losing weight with an aim to attain the thin model. It is good to note that being underweight presents health concerns to a woman as being overweight can.

FACTORS AFFECTING WEIGHT

Two major factors that affect eight are:

(1) Genes.

(2) Hormones.

Other contributory factors are lifestyle, activity level etc.

GENERAL SCREENING TOOLS

These give a fair idea whether a person is underweight, overweight or has a healthy weight. Using different tools in combination gives a better categorization of a person's weight.

(1) BMI (Body Mass Index)

This is a tool used to categorize tissue mass in an individual.

It is the weight in kilograms divided by a square of the height in metres.

$$BMI = \frac{Weight \ (kg)}{Height \ (metres) \times Height \ (metres)}$$

For examples, Mrs. A weights 80kg and has a height of 1.6m

$$BM \ 1 = \frac{80}{1.6 \times 1.6} = \frac{80}{2.56}$$

$$= 31.25$$

CLASSIFICATION FOR BODY MASS INDEX (BMI)

WEIGHT CATEGORIES	BMI (kg/m^2
Under weight	<18.5
Healthy weight	$18.5 - 24.9$
Over weight	$25 - 29.9$
Obese (Class I)	$30 - 34.9$
Severely Obese (Class II)	$35 - 39.9$
Morbidly Obese (Class III)	$40 - 49.9$
Super Obese (Class III)	>50

(2) MEASUREMENT OF WAIST CIRCUMFERENCE

The waist is key because tummy fat can be serious and increases risk of Type 2 Diabetes Mellitus, High Blood pressure and heart disease.

It is done by applying a measuring tape around the waist at the level of the navel.

Ensure you breathe out before reading the measurement for accuracy.

WOMEN should not be greater than 35inches

MEN should not be greater than 40inches.

(3) WAIST TO HIP RATIO

This is done by measuring the thinnest part of the waist, and dividing it by the widest part of the hip.

HEALTHY: It should not be greater than 0.85 in women. It should not be greater than 0.9 in men.

PROBLEMS OF OVERWEIGHT

This increases risk of certain diseases such as heart disease, diabetes and osteoarthritis.

WHAT TO DO

- Healthy eating.

- Increase physical activity.

LOW WEIGHT(UNDERWEIGHT)

A low weight can pose serious problems to a woman's health. This could occur as a result of the following:

- Family history: This refers to genetic make up.

- A high metabolism: This will break down food faster than rate of intake.
- Frequent physical activity: This may burn significant amount of calories.

- Physical illness or chronic disease: This can lead to losses through vomiting or diarrhoea, reduced intake due to low appetite. Illnesses that can lead to significant drop in weight include cancer, thyroid disorders, digestive conditions etc.
- Mental illness: Depression and anxiety can significantly affect one's ability to eat.

PROBLEMS ASSOCIATED WITH UNDERWEIGHT.

The complications of underweight are mostly due to the underlying cause which is malnutrition.

(1) Decrease in immune function.

(2) Increased risk of osteoporosis.

(3) Menstrual dysfunction : This includes irregular menses or absent menses as a result of anovulation which can ultimately lead to infertility.

(4) Increased risk of preterm delivery in pregnant women.

(5) Hair loss, hair thinning and dryness of the skin.

WHAT TO DO

(1) Take smaller frequent meals with snacks between meals.

(2) Take nutrient- rich meals such as whole grains, diary products, nuts and seeds.

(3) Avoid caffeine and alcohol.

(4) Exercise: Yes! Exercise adds muscle to the body and stimulate appetite.

CHAPTER 8

SUPPLEMENTATION

- Dietary Supplements are products taken orally (by mouth) and contain ingredients intended to supplement one's diet.

- Nutrient compounds in supplements includes Vitamins, Minerals, Fibre, Fatty Acids and Amino Acids.

- Formulations can be in form of pill, capsule, tablets, or liquid.

Women at different stages of life have different biological needs.

Supplements help to boost nutrition and fill up nutrition gaps.

Note: Supplements are not mandatory if one's diet is optimal, meeting the need for minerals and vitamins.

Consult a doctor before using a supplement to know which is best for you.

SUPPLEMENT	INDICATION/FUNCTION	DIETARY SOURCES
FOLIC ACID	- Child – bearing years - Pre – pregnancy -During pregnancy/ Breastfeeding **FUNCTION:** - Support Brain health and cell reproduction. - Reduce risk of birth defects of brain or spinal cord.	Legumes: beans, peas, Green Vegetables, Beets, Citrus fruits, nuts and seeds. Beef liver, papaya, banana, Avocado, grains.
IRON	- Women in their 30's - Pregnant women - Women with moderate to heavy menstrual flow. **FUNCTION:** For production of healthy red blood cells.	Shell Fish E.G Shrimps, Prawns. Organ Meat: Liver, Legumes: Beans, Red meat, turkey, dark chocolate.
VITAMIN B COMPLEX	Pre-menopausal and post-menopausal women. **FUNCTION:** - Improves mood, digestion, sleep and energy. - Support hair, skin and nail health	Whole grains, fruits/vegetables B12 – Meat, Fish & Milk

ANTI—OXIDANTS (VITAMIN C & E)	**FUNCTION:** - Support healthy skin - Vitamin C boost immune system.	Vitamin C — fruits e.g Lemons, paw-paw, oranges. Vitamin E — Almonds, peanuts, avocado, mango, snail, crayfish.
FISH OIL	Women in their 40's (peri-menopausal) **FUNCTION:** - Support heart and brain health	Mackerel, Cod liver oil, sardines, soya beans.
VITAMIN D & CALCIUM	Women in their 50's (peri-menopausal) **FUNCTION:** - Promote bone health	Diary: Milk, yoghurt, cheese. Non diary: Sea food, leafy greens, dried fruit, legumes. Vitamin D: Sunlight, egg yolk, mushroom.

CHAPTER 9

VACCINATION

Vaccination is an effective way of preventing a number of infectious diseases.

- Schedules may differ from one country to another.

- Ask your health care professional what vaccinations are available for women and the specified schedule.

VACCINE	DISEASE	DATE	
HPV	Human papilloma Virus	Dose	1 - - - - 2 - - - - 3 - - - -
HBV	Hepatitis B virus	Dose	1 - - - - 2 - - - - 3 - - - -
TT (TETANUS TOXOID)	Tetanus		1 - - - - 2 - - - - 3 - - - - 4 - - - - 5 - - - - Booster Dose - - -

Note:

- HPV is recommended for young women before first sexual contact and protects against cervical cancer.

- Hepatitis B vaccine is particularly important for health care workers and women with multiple sex partners.

- Five doses of T. T (Tetanus Toxoid) with booster does given every 10years confers life immunity. First dose can be started in pregnancy.

HEALTH SCREENING

Health screening entails looking for disease before symptoms appear. It helps to detect diseases easily for prompt intervention.

- Screening Tests required will depend on a woman's age, family history of disease conditions and her risk factors for certain diseases.

SCREENING	FREQUENCY	RESULT
BREAST EXAMINATION	Self- examination: Monthly Professional examination yearly	
BLOOD PRESSURE	Yearly	
BLOOD GLUCOSE	Yearly	
BLOOD CHOLESTEROL	Yearly	
PAP SMEAR	Yearly	
MAMMOGRAM	Every other year from age 40	

CHAPTER 10

SEX

Sex is an intimate contact between partners, primarily designed for procreation but is also a source of pleasure and relaxation.

THE SEXUAL RESPONSE CYCLE

This refers to the sequence of physical and emotional changes that occur during sex. Knowing how the body responds during the different phases can enhance one's sexual experience and improve relationship with a partner.

A common model by Masters and Kaplan, describes four phases of the sexual response cycle.

NOTE: This is a general guide and may vary among individuals.

(1) DESIRE (LIBIDO)

Consists of sexual urges, fantasies and wishes.

CHARACTERISTICS:

- Increase in muscle tension.

- Increased breathing and heart rate.

- Nipples harden and become erect.

- Breast fullness.

- Swelling of the clitoris, labia minora and vaginal walls due to increased blood flow to genitals.

- Vaginal lubrication.

(2) EXCITEMENT (AROUSAL)

- Changes in phase 1 intensifies.

- The clitoris become sensitive and retracts to avoid direct stimulation.

- Muscle spasm in feet, face and hands.

(3) ORGASM (CLIMAX):

- Also called Climax, this is the peak of sexual pleasure.

- It is the shortest phase and last for a few seconds.

- Involuntary muscle contractions.

- Higher increase in Breathing, heart rate and blood pressure.

- Muscle spasm in feet.

- Sudden forceful release of sexual tension.

- Contraction of muscles of the vagina and uterus.

(4) RESOLUTION.

The body slowly returns to its normal level of function.

- Swelling reduces.

- It is marked by a general sense of well-being and often, fatigue.

NOTE: Women can rapidly return to the orgasm phase with further stimulation, leading to multiple orgasms.

HEALTH BENEFITS OF SEX

1. Improves heart health.

2. Lowers blood pressure.

3. Strengthens muscles.

4. Burns calories.

5. Boost immune system.

6. Improves sleep.

7. Relieves pain due to release of oxytocin (the feel good hormone).

8. Reduces stress and anxiety.

9. Boost self esteem.

10. Improve fertility.

SAFE SEX

This entails protecting oneself and partner from sexually transmitted infections.

1. Use protection if not in a monogamous relationship.

2. Get tested for sexually transmitted infections (STI) regularly.

3. Seek prompt treatment for sexually transmitted infections.

Note: Oral sex is not completely safe as assumed.

Infections like herpes, syphilis, hepatitis B, gonorrhea and human papilloma virus (HPV) can be transmitted through oral sex.

SEXUAL DYSFUNCTION

(1) Problem of desire (LOW LIBIDO)

This refers to a low interest in sexual activity.

CAUSES

1. Medication such as Antidepressants.

2. Chronic medical condition such as Diabetes, heart disease.

3. Hormonal changes: this may be due to pregnancy, breast feeding or menopause.

4. Anxiety or depression.

5. Stress and Fatigue.

6. Boredom with regular sexual routines.

(2) PROBLEM OF AROUSAL

The inability to be physically aroused could be due to any of the following:

- Anxiety.

- Inadequate stimulation.

- Poor vaginal lubrication.

(3) PAINFUL SEX

This is known as dyspareunia.

Causes include:

- Sexually transmitted Infections.

- Pelvic mass such as fibroids.

- Vaginitis.

- Poor lubrication.

- Vaginismus (spasm of muscles surrounding the vaginal entrance). This could occur as a result of sexual phobia or fear and previous trauma.

- Endometriosis (uterine tissue growing elsewhere).

(4) Lack of Orgasm (Anorgasmia)

This refers to the absence of sexual climax (orgasm)

Causes include:

- A woman's sexual inhibition.

- Psychological factors such as past sexual trauma or abuse.

- Inexperience.

- Medications.

- Chronic diseases.

- Insufficient stimulation.

MAKING SEX BETTER

1. Kegel's exercise:

Kegel's exercises helps to strengthen pelvic muscles. These are the muscles that support the vagina and surrounding pelvic organs.

Step 1

Identify the muscles: This is done by tightening the muscle used to stop urine flow midstream.

Step 2

Hold the contraction for 2-3 seconds then release.

Repeat this 10 times. Do 5 sets a day.

NOTE: Kegel can be done anywhere, anytime and in any position.

2. DIET

Take foods rich in Vitamin C.

Ensure adequate water intake.

3. LUBRICANTS

Use water based lubricants for vaginal dryness and to enhance lubrication.

CHAPTER 11

HEALTHY RELATIONSHIP

The quality of your relationships can affect various aspects of your health: mental health, physical health and can influence lifestyle. Good relationships improve one's health and wellbeing.

QUALITIES OF HEALTHY RELATIONSHIPS

- Free communication without judgment.

- Trust and respect.

- Engagement in healthy activities.

- Honesty.

- Independence.

- Compassion.

- Loyalty.

EFFECTS OF HEALTHY RELATIONSHIP

1. Reduces stress.

2. Improves quality of life.

3. Reduces risk of mental health issues such as depression.

4. Encourages healthy behavior and lifestyle.

5. Improves healing and recovery from ailments.

6. Improves heart health.

THE FIVE (5) LOVE LANGUAGES

These concepts of love language were developed by Gary chapman PhD, a renowned marriage therapist.

It is common to feel unloved when you don't receive love in a language you understand.

Knowing your love language and understanding that of your partner will improve your relationship.

Study these five love languages with illustrations:

1. Words of affirmation: Example 'I love you.'

2. Acts of service: Rendering exceptional services.

3. Gifts: Even little gifts can speak volumes.

4. Quality time: Features a need for attention.

5. Physical touch : Such as hugs, sex.

A NOTE ON VIOLENCE

- Gender based violence is a global issue.

- The most common are battering and sexual assault in which women are the victims.

- Most acts of violence against women are carried out by close persons.

Note: most cases of battering begin with verbal threat and abuse.

WHAT TO DO

1. Tell a friend, family member, clergy, health professional.

2. Watch out for warning signs such as threats.

3. Have a ready-made exit plan in case of an emergency.

4. Identify help centers.

Note: Many cases of violence against women are concealed for reasons of fear and shame.

Women must be encouraged to speak out early and seek help.

CHAPTER 12

Frequently Asked Questions (FAQs)

1. Is my menstrual cycle normal?

Menstrual cycles are different for each person. A typical menstrual cycle will last for 28 days, but cycle lengths between 21-35days is considered normal, and a menstrual flow for 2-8days.

2. How should a healthy vagina smell?

The vagina has a natural smell that is not offensive.

While diet, hygiene and other factors may affect the smell of a woman's vagina, any significant change in odour should be reported. A fishy smell suggests a bacterial infection while a bread-like smell suggests a yeast infection.

3. Can vaginal itching be normal?

Yes. Hormonal changes that lower estrogen levels such as right before a period could cause thinning of vaginal skin making it dry, irritated and itchy.

Consult with a doctor if you experience severe itching.

4. What is the difference between sexually transmitted diseases (STD) and sexually transmitted infections (STI)?

Both terms are frequently used interchangeably but here is the difference: Sexually transmitted infections don't necessary mean symptoms are present, most people with STI are without symptoms. But in sexually transmitted diseases, symptoms are present.

5. Why do I have facial hair?

It's normal to get more facial hair with aging but a sudden change in facial hair suggests hormonal imbalance. Other causes include use of steroids or oral contraceptive pills, polycystic ovarian syndrome etc.

6.What causes breast to sag?

With age, the ligaments that support breast tissue lose their elasticity. Also, any condition that causes breast to enlarge and then shrink such as weight gain and loss, pregnancy and breast feeding will lead to sagging as the skin does not snap back.

7. How do I prevent Yeast infection?

Yeast thrives in warm, damp places. It is important to wear loose breathable underwear such as cotton, and allow the vagina to breathe from time to time by going underwear-free. Other measures include avoiding the use of soap and other chemicals on vaginal skin which will disrupt vaginal PH, destroy natural bacteria and lead to an overgrowth of fungi.

8.Can I have sex during pregnancy?

Sex during pregnancy is safe as the baby is protected by a cervical mucus plug which prevents entry of substances from the vagina into the womb. However, consult with a doctor if you have a history of previous miscarriage or preterm labour.

9. Can I become pregnant during breast feeding?

Yes.' Exclusive' breast feeding offers contraception by suppressing ovulation, but take note that ovulation will occur before the first menstrual period. It is advisable to use birth control.

10. What is the best method of contraception?

There is no 'best' method of contraception as the best method is different for every woman, can change over time and depends on several factors. Consider the following when making a choice and talk to a health professional.

- Overall state of health.

- Desire to have children now or in the future.

- A need to prevent sexually transmitted infections.

- Personal preferences.

- Compliance.

REFRENCES

Cathy, Cassata: 10 Amazing facts about your breast, breast 2019

Zoldan, Rachael: 20 Amazing facts all women should know, 2007

Mayo Clinic Staff: Menopause – Symptoms and causes, 2017

www.breastcancer.org: Breast Self-Exam, 2018

ABOUT THE AUTHOR

Dr Felicitas Ud, a seasoned medical practitioner and wellness coach is passionate about teaching and motivating people -children, women, men to take charge of their health and wellness.

She is the founder and CEO, Well Group Nigeria, an organization that is transforming lives through healthy living.

www.ingramcontent.com/pod-product-compliance
Lightning Source LLC
Chambersburg PA
CBHW051356280526
45784CB00007B/2980